The 28 Day Intermittent Fasting Diet Weight Loss Program

Feel Stronger, Leaner, and Healthier than ever before!

Table of Contents

Introduction

I want to thank you and congratulate you for purchasing the book, *"The 28 Day Intermittent Fasting Diet Weight Loss Program: Feel Stronger, Leaner, and Healthier than ever before!"*.

This book has actionable information on how to follow intermittent fasting to lose weight, become healthier, feel stronger and leaner.

Intermittent fasting is undoubtedly one of the most effortless and painless ways of losing weight. Think about it; all you need to do is perhaps skip a meal here and there (which most of us do anyway whenever we are very busy) to lose weight. It sounds too good to be true but the truth is that it does work. And there are tons of success stories out there to prove that it does work.

However, you have to do is right (i.e. while following guidelines that will support you throughout your weight loss journey) if you really want to achieve sustainable weight loss.

And lucky for you, this book has information that you can follow to make that a reality. The book will teach you the ins and outs of intermittent fasting as well as how to put it in action.

It even provides a daily plan that you can follow to follow intermittent fasting for a month.

Let's begin.

Thanks again for purchasing this book. I hope you enjoy it!

A Comprehensive Background to Intermittent Fasting

What Is Intermittent Fasting

In simple terms, intermittent fasting is simply refers to a way of eating where you alternate/cycle between periods of voluntary fasting and periods of eating/feasting.

The fasting may be done for as long as a few hours to days depending on the type of intermittent fasting method employed. Intermittent fasting puts more focus on WHEN followers eat as opposed to WHAT its followers eat. It is about how long you are required to space out the time between one meal and the next one. This means it is not like a conventional diet that prescribes that to eat and what you should avoid. This makes intermittent fasting, not a diet, but a **dieting pattern.**

With this eating pattern, what you need to do is to go without ingesting any calorie rich food or drink long enough so that you get your body to expend dietary calories within the body (from the food you eat), as this forces it to start burning stored energy from glycogen and fats. Your ultimate goal is to get the body to actually start burning fat. Well, you don't just fast aimlessly; you have to fast while following the guidelines provided in the different fasting methods that have been developed. However, at bare minimum, you should give your body about 12-14 hours to get into a state where it burns stored body fat for energy if you want to benefit from intermittent fasting. You can do more; up to 36 hours if you want to push yourself and can do it.

The question is; why are we doing all this? What's the logic/explanation behind going without eating anything for at least 12-14 hours?

Let me explain that in detail:

How Does Intermittent Fasting Work?

To best understand how intermittent fasting works, it is important to understand how the body uses the food you eat as is goes through 2 main states, namely the fed state and the fasted state.

How The Body Uses The Food You Eat

When you eat, your body will spend the next 3-5 hours digesting the food you've eaten into small absorbable molecules and then absorbing the molecules into the bloodstream where they can be transported to different parts of the body. These molecules are glucose from the breakdown of carbohydrates, fatty acids from the breakdown of fats and amino acids from the breakdown of proteins. Considering the fact that much of the typical American diet is high in carbohydrates, it means that you essentially have high amounts of glucose being produced from the breakdown of carbohydrates. When the glucose is absorbed into the bloodstream, this means the blood glucose levels increase, something that the pancreas detects after which it secretes insulin from the beta cells. Insulin plays a very important role of glucose regulation. It does that by signaling the cells, through the insulin receptors that every cell has, to open up in order to take up glucose. Insulin will keep the cells open as long as there is glucose in the bloodstream. However, the cells have their limits as far as how much glucose they can use is concerned. So when this limit is reached, they become less sensitive to insulin, something that automatically makes the liver more sensitive to insulin. Insulin in this case signals the liver to convert glucose into glycogen, which is stored within the liver and muscle cells. The structure of glycogen molecules allows them to stack perfectly on each other to fit compactly. That's why they are easily stored in the cells of the muscles and the liver.

These glycogen stores fill up pretty fast though as they can only store up to 2000kcal of energy at a time so the body has to find an alternative storage area. The fat stores around the body are a perfect storage area in such cases. Since these stores can only store fat, the body is forced to convert any excess glucose into fatty acids and glycerol, a process known as de novo lipogenesis. In Latin, the breakdown is as follows: De means from, novo means new, lipo means fat and genesis means creation. Combine them all together and it will read 'creation of fat from new.

A small portion of this fat is stored around the liver but the rest of it is transported and deposited in different body parts. Unlike in the production of glycogen and its storage in the liver, there is NO LIMIT in the production and storage of fat in the body through the process of de novo lipogenesis. If we are constantly in the fed state and consuming more calories than our bodies require, then the fatty tissues keep accumulating all around the body. In due course, we put on more weight over time and become overweight or obese.

This entire process takes about 8-12 hours and results to depletion of dietary glucose from the bloodstream. During all this time, since the last meal, you are considered to be in the fed state, which is categorized into the absorptive state and the post absorptive state. If you don't eat anything, your body starts a very interesting process to survive. This process entails getting into the fasted state.

The Fasted State

The fasted state is when the body starts 'eating' what it already stored in the glycogen stores and the fat stores.

The process takes place with the help of another hormone produced by the alpha cells of the pancreas known as glucagon. Glucagon is only produced when insulin levels fall and when the concentrations of dietary blood glucose are very low in a bid to help the body to meet its immediate (short term) energy demands.

So how exactly does the process work?

Well, when the pancreas detects reduced blood glucose levels coupled with low insulin concentrations in the bloodstream, it releases glucagon. The role of glucagon is to signal the liver to metabolize the available glycogen into glucose, which is then transported through the bloodstream to different parts of the body. The newly made glucose is used just as the dietary glucose. However, since glycogen reserves are limited, the body soon finds itself needing more energy to keep going. And it does solve the problem by signaling the fat stores around the body to release the fat (in form of triglycerides) through the bloodstream- towards the liver) where the fats are broken down into fatty acids and glycerol. These then go through a series of metabolic processes that end up producing energy molecules referred to as ketones in a process known as ketosis. The body is able to run on these fully, especially because ketones, just as glucose, can cross the blood brain barrier.

Note: The glycogen stored away in the muscle and liver cells are usually sufficient to supply the rest of the body with glucose for a period ranging from one day to a day and a half before they are depleted completely. Beyond this point, the body now starts to run exclusively on its fat reserves (ketones) as fuel.

Well, I am not saying that you will have to fast for 36 hours to burn fat; your body starts burning fat long before it exhausts its glycogen reserves. The process takes place with the help of other hormones such as the human growth hormone.

It is a pity that most of us are constantly feeding every few hours meaning that we are always in the fed state. We are used to eating 3 large meals a day or 6 small ones and a lot of snacking in between. In short, your body only uses the incoming food energy and NEVER gets an opportunity to utilize its ever-piling energy reserves.

And that is why we are continually putting on weight and finding it extremely difficult to lose it no matter the effort put in. Why? Because you are too afraid to give your digestive system a break, which your body would greatly benefit from.

I know you might be thinking; isn't going without food for an extended period unhealthy? Well, absolutely not and I will explain:

How Intermittent Fasting Has Evolved

Intermittent fasting is an ancient practice that has been part of the human nature since the very beginning of time. Food was not always readily available like it is now.

The body of the early man had to store food energy as body fat to maintain life and endure the tough times. If early man never developed this adaptive mechanism of efficient storage and retrieval process of food energy, the human race would have been wiped away from the face of earth many centuries ago.

The moment when food became more available, many human religions and cultures were already prescribing periods of fasting. For instance, Jesus is believed to have fasted for 40 days and 40 nights. Subsequently those who proclaim the Christian faith do undertake themselves voluntary periods of fasting without any signs of significant health damage. Likewise, the Muslims also fast during the holy month of Ramadhan. They also fast two times a week on a regular basis during the rest of the year.

Fasting Is Not Starvation

Most people usually don't understand the difference between starving and fasting yet the two turn out to be very far apart.

So what is the difference?

Starvation is a situation where you completely lack anything to eat against your will. It is the deficiency of nutrients that are necessary to maintain life of a living organism. In such a scenario, the organism will slowly become emaciated and eventually die. Starvation is not deliberate and it is something you cannot control. When you starve, you usually have no idea when you will have your next meal. Actually, it may not even arrive at all.

Fasting, on the other hand, as you've read before is the controlled and voluntary abstinence of any sort of food. It is done 100% on purpose. It's also perfectly orchestrated meaning that you plan to do it yourself either because religion demands that you do so, because of its health benefits or due to whatever other reasons.

Fasting In Everyday Life

Fasting is actually a part of your everyday life. For instance, did you know that you fast every night in your sleep? Actually, this is how the English word 'breakfast' came to be. Breakfast simply means 'breaking the fast' with a morning meal after some ten or twelve hours when you had your last meal. The fact that you sleep through the greater part of your fast makes it quite painless.

Fasting is so critical and beneficial that animals do it whenever they are sick. Haven't you noticed how you and other people lose appetite whenever you are sick? This perhaps explains why fasting has been referred to as the physician within.

Against the persistent onslaught of media ads that taunt your innate and primitive urge to eat as often as you can (whenever food is available so that you store some for a rainy day- which in most cases never comes), willpower these days is in short supply. "Are you hungry? Grab a hot dog for only 99 cents". Every hour, you are interrupted by a boisterous disruption that requires your gustatory attentiveness.

We now live in a world where everybody is eating all the time. It has even come to a point where it is difficult to tell when we should eat. As it is for most of us, having 3 meals a day i.e. breakfast, lunch and dinner has become more of a cultural artifact than it is a biological necessity. As it turns out, the modern man is not only eating more than he has ever had; but crucially more often than he ever has.

This habit of feeding from dusk to dawn is the reason why a large portion of the human population is struggling with constant weight gain, insulin resistance and diseases. That's why you should make fasting your first priority. However, as you adopt intermittent fasting, it is good to be prepared psychologically for the changes. Your body is already accustomed to eating too often and will 'resist' your conscious action to not eat as often through all manner of responses some of which we will discuss next.

Dealing With the "Side Effects" Of Intermittent Fasting

If you are just getting started to intermittent fasting, it is normal to experience some mild side effects although they soon subside. Just as a registered dietician Stephanie Ferrari once said:

"Think about it this way - people don't go from potato couch to tri-athlete overnight. Your body needs to acclimatize to any extreme changes. So you're going to experience some side effects when you suddenly stop eating for long periods of time."

At first, these side effects may seem unbearable, but knowing how to deal with them will go a long way in helping you reap all the benefits.

1. Hunger pangs

The most obvious side effect is hunger. If you have conditioned your body to eat five or six times every day, then it expects food at specific times. Ghrelin, also known as 'hunger hormone, is produced and secreted by the stomach. Its function is to stimulate appetite when the stomach is empty. Other than that, it is also responsible for promoting fat storage and increases food intake.

The more hours you fast, the more the levels of ghrelin continue to increase and thus, the hungrier you become. At the beginning, you will need your sheer willpower. But the 3rd and 5th days of following intermittent fasting regularly will bring out the worst since this is the period when ghrelin secretion is at its peak. However, it comes a time when you are ready to break your fast and you are not even hungry.

So how do you effectively combat such extreme hunger pangs during the first few days? A weight loss and nutrition specialist Dr. Luiza Petre suggests that you drink plenty of water to keep your belly full and help satisfy that nasty urge of putting something in your mouth. Within 30 minutes of waking up, glug down at least a liter of water. Later on, as much as feel like eating, drink some more water before your meals. Read more here about the importance of water when on a fast.

2. Feeling cold

Your body and especially the fingers and toes are going to feel cold when fasting. If it happens, don't freak out, as this happens for a reason.

You are colder because no heat is being produced from the digestive muscle work that takes place when you eat frequently. To combat this issue, put on warm clothing (put on gloves or socks if necessary), take a warm shower, be active even if that means taking a walk to help the blood circulation moving all over and lastly, sip hot non-sweetened beverages such as coffee or tea.

3. Constipation, bloating and heartburn

The lining of your stomach produces acid to help digest ingested food. Your body will still be used to your old eating patterns so the stomach releases the acid at certain times. Even after you begin your fasting regimen, chances are your body will still stick to your previous eating behaviours. That means that, even when the stomach is empty, you may experience some heartburn.

This side effect should disappear with time as your body adjusts to the new eating patterns. Therefore, keep drinking water and when you are about to eat, avoid spicy and greasy foods as these could make your heartburn even worse. If the heartburn persists, seek advice from your doctor.

You may also become constipated when fasting and this may cause bloat and discomfort. Drinking plenty of water is the perfect solution to this problem.

4. Low energy and reduction in athletic performance

When fasting, your body does not get the constant source of energy it used to get when eating all day. It is no surprise then that you'll expect to feel a bit sluggish inside the first few weeks of your new fasting regimen.

Therefore, you'll want to keep your day as relaxed as possible to exert the minimum amount of energy. If you exercise regularly, you might consider giving your body a break or just perform some light exercises such as yoga or walking. It's also important to get plenty of sleep.

5. Irritability or feeling 'hangry'

An extended period of hunger can have some emotional consequences. According to the Merriam Webster dictionary, the word 'hangry' is a clever blend word of 'hungry' and 'angry'.

It is therefore used to describe a person's tendency to become irritable due to hunger. To deal with this, you need to stay away from people or situations that are likely to irritate you more. Instead, keep yourself busy or focus on the things that make you happy.

6. Headaches

A migraine or headache that comes about as a result of intermittent fasting may not always be caused by a drop in the blood sugar levels. They can be triggered by the stress hormones produced by the body when in the fasted state. More often than not, they are also caused by dehydration and inadequate sleep. This is why you are encouraged to drink plenty of water and get enough rest.

With what you've learned in mind, let's now discuss the specific steps you should take to follow intermittent fasting with impressive results.

Step 1: Decide Which Intermittent Fasting Method/Protocol To Use

There are many ways to practice intermittent fasting. Basically, the most popular and easy ways of performing IF involves taking advantage of your natural 'overnight fast'. In other words, this means skipping breakfast then breaking the fast a few hours later during the day. Normally, when you've gone more than 12 hours from dinner the previous night without food, you are undoubtedly in the fasted state and this is the period when your body relies entirely on stored fat for fuel.

You can choose any of the following fasting protocols/methods:

1: The Leangains protocol also known as 16:8 diet

Developed by bodybuilder Martin Berkhan, the 16:8 dieting pattern is by far the most popular protocol. It entails fasting for 16 hours and dedicating the rest of the time i.e. 8 hours for eating.

So how do you go about executing the 16:8 method? Well, you could skip breakfast every day such that you take the first meal of your day during the lunch hour. Basically, you don't take breakfast when you wake up but you eat lunch and dinner as you would normally within an 8 hour window. Therefore, the idea is to fast overnight plus the first 6 hours of the day. In total, you will have fasted for 16 hours and then dedicated the remaining 8 hours to eating.

For instance, if you wake up every day at 7:00 a.m., you will be required to skip breakfast and not eat anything for the next six hours. That means you will have your lunch at 1.00 p.m. and then dinner at 9.00pm; you may snack any time between this eating window although it is best if you consolidate all the calories into the 2 main meals. This 16:8 split i.e. 16 hours of fasting and 8 hours of eating should be carried out on a daily basis.

It is important to keep a constant daily feeding pattern. This is due of the <u>hormonal entrainment</u> of the meal patterns. Ghrelin hormone is an appetite stimulant. Studies show that the stomach tells the brain when to eat. Therefore, when you establish a regular schedule of your meals, your stomach regulates the secretion of ghrelin so that you won't experience hunger pangs as you fast.

2: Eat stop eat

Bodybuilder Brad Pilon developed this method of fasting. It involves fasting for a full 24 hours for 2 non-consecutive days every week.

For example, assume that dinner is the last meal you had at exactly 9.00 p.m. You are required to fast overnight and the entire day that follows. That means skipping breakfast and lunch so that you may break your fast again at exactly 9:00 p.m.

This method of fasting is not that easy and that is why it is only recommended to be carried out for only 2 non-consecutive days. However, by the time you complete the 24 hours of fasting, your body will have reached a very deep level of fat oxidation and lipolysis while insulin levels will be very low and this is quite desirable.

You may be thinking that such a fast may cause you to binge on food when you break your fast to an extent that the benefits of the previous day's fast will be negated. However, that is not true. Sure, you may eat a lot of calories the following day but still the calories you consume will not come anywhere close to what you would have consumed if you were eating normally for the 2 days. This means you will still be left with a huge caloric deficit even when you binge-eat the day after you fast.

3: ADF - Alternate day fasting (fasting every other day)

Just as the name suggests, you are required to alternate between one day of eating and then eating very little on the next day. Dr. Johnson, the mastermind behind this method of fasting came up with the protocol after inspiration from a 2003 study. In the study, mice registered outstanding improvements in weight loss when fed every other day (on alternate days).

On the fasting day, you are supposed to consume 20% of your total daily energy expenditure. That makes it 400 and 500 calories for women and men respectively per day given that the recommended daily calorie intake is 2000 and 2500 respectively.

How fast you adapt to this protocol depends on factors such as your blood pressure and cholesterol levels, weight and how insulin resistant you are. If you strictly adhere to this dieting pattern, you can effectively lose between 1 to 2 pounds (453 – 907 grams) of body weight every week.

4: The Warrior Diet

Ori Hofmekler popularized this method of fasting. It involves fasting during the better part of the day, then squeezing all your calories in the evening. The main aim here is to skip breakfast and lunch then 'feast' on a huge dinner within a 4 hour window at the end of the day. Basically, this is a 20:4 hour split. 20 hours of fasting and 4 hours of feasting.

The advantage with this method is that it allows you to eat a very large and satiating meal at the end of the day. Therefore, it is most suitable for you if you had plans to go out to dinner with friends or family, where plenty of calories of food might be involved. During the feasting period, you should start the meal course with vegetables, then proteins and finally fats in that order. You may then fill what space is left with carbs.

Ori Hofmekler intentionally refers to the 4-hour window as the 'overeating' period. He believes that human beings are nocturnal eaters. In other words, humans are programmed to eat only at night. Moreover, he believes that the reason why the feast should only be at night is to make the most of the ability of the nervous system to enable the body to recover, relax and promote digestion. Feasting at night also stimulates your body to secrete hormones that enable the body to burn more fat when working during the day.

The downside is that fasting for this long during the day might be a bit challenging and may take some time to get used to. However, once you get to grips with the method, it leads you to a deep level of 'fat adaptation' and low insulin.

5: Spontaneous Meal Skipping

Sometimes you just don't need to follow any structured intermittent fasting protocol to lose weight. You may decide to miss some meals from time to time depending on the period that is convenient for you. For example, if you are too busy or if you are not hungry, then you don't have to bother yourself preparing or ordering food.

If you wake up one morning before heading to work and don't feel like eating, you could always skip breakfast entirely and wait for lunch or dinner. If you skip a meal you feel inclined to, you will basically be doing spontaneous fasts. That shouldn't be a problem as your body is very well equipped to handle long periods of drought and famine, let alone missing a meal or two every now and then.

N.B: No matter which fasting protocol you follow, make sure you avoid eating or drinking any calories when fasting. Be keen to avoid things such as chewing gums, sweetened drinks etc.

You can choose the fasting protocol that you feel best suits your circumstances. For a complete beginner, the 16:8 fasting protocol is the best to start with. To make your fast effective, move to step 2.

Step 2: Calculate Your Calorie Intake

Do you know how many calories you should consume during the fasting window? This is one of the most common questions beginners ask when they want to get started with the IF regimen. So if you want to know how many calories you should consume to lose weight and enjoy other benefits, you'll have to do so with the help of this calculator.

Claims that you don't need to watch your calorie intake when practicing IF are absolutely false and baseless, especially if you really want to see results, fast. If you are serious about maximizing on the healing and weight loss powers of intermittent fasting, you will have to learn about creating an energy balance and a caloric deficit.

Calorie deficit

When you consume fewer calories than your body uses up, then you put your body in a calorie deficit situation, which is also known as an energy deficit. If you are fasting with the intention of losing weight, then you will have to expose your body to a sustained calorie deficit that is just sufficient to have a significant impact on your weight. But again, you have to be careful to limit the deficit because if it is very huge, it may present you with unnecessary physiological and health problems.

For example, slashing your calorie intake to 50% of your <u>Total Daily Energy Expenditure</u> would definitely have the desired effect on your body i.e. a significant reduction in your body fat levels. However, that would also cause you a lot of problems such as bone frailty, immunosuppression, mood disturbances, muscle loss and metabolic adaptation among others.

So what is the right way to create a calorie deficit without harming your health? Let the deficit be slight but also big enough to have a considerable impact on weight loss. For instance, if you were to consume about 90% of your <u>Total Daily Energy Expenditure</u>, weight loss would be certain to take place but slightly slower over time. However, you wouldn't experience any of the negative side effects mentioned above.

Energy balance

Energy balance is the relationship between the calories your body consumes against the calories it expends.

With this in mind, the scientifically indisputable truth is summed up in the following phrase; that *'significant weight loss requires you to use up more calories than you consume'*.

This means that *if you consume extra calories than your body expends, the pendulum swings to the positive side of the energy balance.* **Positive energy balance** is the term used when the body fat levels increase since the surplus energy has to be converted and stored as fat.

On the other hand, *if you consume less calories than your body expends, the pendulum swings to the negative side of the energy balance.* **Negative energy balance** is the term used when there is a reduction in your body fat levels in consequence of the calorie deficit created after your body burns fat as fuel.

Let's take this even further by discussing macronutrients.

Step 3: Calculate The Macronutrient Intake

Macronutrients are the main nutrients that constitute the food you eat. They are what your body requires in relatively large amounts to grow, survive and even reproduce. That said, there are 3 macronutrients that your body can't live without. These are proteins, carbohydrates and fats.

When on an intermittent fasting regimen, you have to know the exact ratio and amounts of the three macronutrients your body needs in order to lose weight effectively.

Generally, the best food for weight loss is that which sates your appetite the most while also supplying your body with plenty of micronutrients and also being relatively low on calories.

Proteins

If you wish to be leaner i.e. lose fat and gain muscle (or lose fat without reducing muscle mass), you will have to emphasize more on your protein intake. By consuming enough proteins while on any IF protocol, your body also tends to recover better from workouts and exercises. Adequate consumption of protein also increases your performance levels in the gym.

How much protein should you consume when breaking your fast? According to research, it is said that you should consume about 0.8 to 1.2 grams of protein for each pound of your body weight each day.

For that reason, if you are obese or overweight, (25% or more in men and 30% or more body fat in women), you need to *consume 1 gram of protein for every pound of your lean body flesh* (fat free mass i.e. flesh, muscle mass bone and water). You need to use a handheld device or a scale to determine your body fat percentage (this simply refers to the percentage of your body weight that comprises fat entirely). For instance, let's assume that you weigh 180 pounds and that 54 pounds of that are made up of fat. This means that your body fat percentage is 30%.

In this case, you should eat (180 - 54) = 126 grams of protein every day.

Fat

Fat is a vital constituent of your diet and assertions that you should take less fat when already struggling to lose weight is a lie. Fat is important for many physiological processes in the body. It plays a huge role in hormone production, nutrient absorption, cell turnover, satiety, insulin sensitivity and muscle growth.

That said fat, should be consumed in moderation to control calorie intake (remember a gram of fat has more than double the amount of calories in carbohydrates and proteins i.e. 9 calories per gram).

In addition, it would be wise to avoid or limit unhealthy fats such as artificial trans-fats (hydrogenated vegetable oil) and saturated fats (fat that is solid at room temperature e.g. meat fat). Instead, consume more of the monounsaturated fats (e.g. peanut, avocado and olive oil) as well as polyunsaturated (omega-6 and omega-3).

According to research, the recommended amount of fat you should consume is *0.3 grams for every pound of your lean body mass*. Thus, if you weigh 180 pounds and your body fat percentage is 30%, your diet should comprise of 100% - 30% = 70% (180 × 0.3) = 37.8 grams of fat.

Carbohydrates

There is a popular belief that you should do away with carbs to stop gaining weight. But that is also a myth. Carbohydrates are important since they're the primary source of fuel when engaging in high intensity exercises, they are the only source of fiber and other micronutrients and can help you gain muscle and strength quicker. If you consume the correct amount of carbs, you will achieve the weight you desire.

By now, you have already established the amount of proteins and fat you need on a daily basis as well as the amount of calories so calculating the amount of carbs will be easy.

1 gram of fat contains 9 calories. 1 gram of carbohydrate and protein both contain about 4 calories each.

To calculate the amount of carbs you need, multiply the amount of protein you should eat by 4 and fat by 9. Calculate the sum of both figures and then subtract the sum from the total calories (Total Daily Energy Expenditure) to get the number of calories from carbohydrates that you remain with. Dividing this amount by 4 will give you the amount of carbs in grams you need to consume daily.

For this example, we'll use the figures we derived from the previous examples;

Fats: 37.8 grams × 9 = 340.2

Proteins: 126 grams × 4 = 504

340.2 + 504 = 844.2

If we assume that your maintenance calories (TDEE) = 1932 calories,

Then 1932 - 844.2 =1087.8 calories remaining for carbohydrates.

1087.8 ÷ 4 = 271.95 grams of carbohydrates per day.

Therefore, your daily macronutrient ratio will be:

Protein - 126 grams

Fats - 37.8 grams

Carbohydrates - 271.95 grams

Let's put everything we've learned into real life practice, let's now discuss how to follow intermittent fasting for 4 weeks to get started.

Step 4: Come Up With A Meal Plan

Now that you have your dietary figures, it is now time to come up with a meal plan. This meal plan will focus on someone following the 16:8 method where they fast from 8pm-12pm and their eating window is between 12pm-8pm. We will also assume that you are only having lunch and dinner; however, if you feel hungry, feel free to have a healthy snack such as some nuts, fruits, smoothies etc.

WEEK 1		
MONDAY	LUNCH	Beef Salad
	DINNER	Cauliflower fried rice
TUESDAY	LUNCH	Previous Night's Leftovers
	DINNER	Chicken Parm Stuffed Peppers
WEDNESDAY	LUNCH	Previous Night's Leftovers
	DINNER	Baked Halibut
THURSDAY	LUNCH	Previous Night's Leftovers

	DINNER	Honey Garlic Glazed Salmon
FRIDAY	LUNCH	Previous Night's Leftovers
	DINNER	Osso Bucco with Soft Polenta
SATURDAY	LUNCH	Previous Night's Leftovers
	DINNER	Pan fried tilapia
SUNDAY	LUNCH	Previous Night's Leftovers
	DINNER	Avocado Chickpea Tuna Salad

To make it easy for you to follow intermittent fasting, you can replicate the above 1-week plan for the entire month. Below are the recipes you can make:

Cauliflower Fried Rice

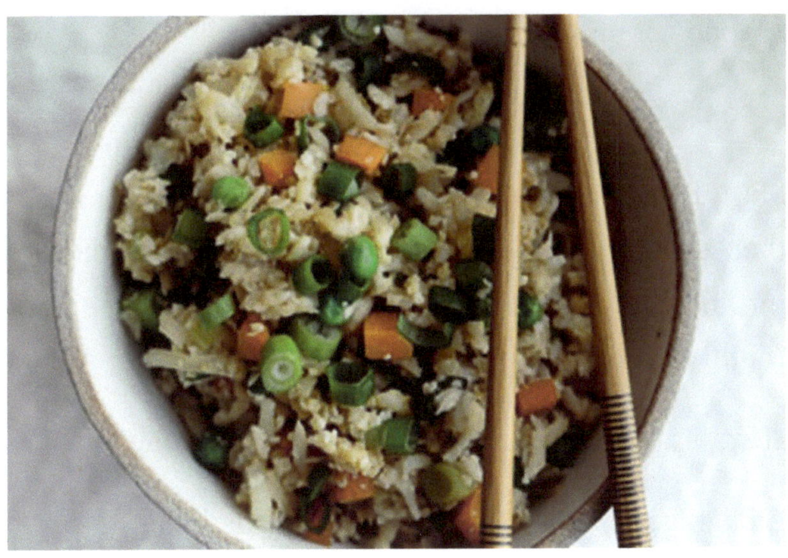

Serves 4

Ingredients

4 sliced scallions with green and white parts separated

2 large eggs

2 garlic cloves, minced

2 tablespoons coconut aminos or tamari

2 tablespoons sesame oil

1 large or 2 to 3 small carrots sliced into small bits

1 medium head of cauliflower

½ cup of frozen peas, thawed

½ diced onion

½ teaspoon of minced ginger

Directions

1. Slice the head of the cauliflower into two equal halves, and then slice off the florets from the stem. Place the florets through the grater of a food processor and process until all cauliflower has been 'riced'.

2. Heat sesame oil in a skillet or huge wok over medium heat.

3. Add ginger, garlic, and sauté for 20 seconds.

4. Stir in the carrots, onions and white parts of the scallions and let it cook for 3 minutes.

5. Add peas and cauliflower rice and stir for another 2 or 3 minutes.

6. Create a well in the middle of the rice and break the eggs inside the well. Stir with a spatula to scramble the eggs.

7. Once the eggs are ready, stir.

8. Finally add the green parts of the scallion and tamari then stir to combine

9. Serve while hot.

Chicken Parm Stuffed Peppers

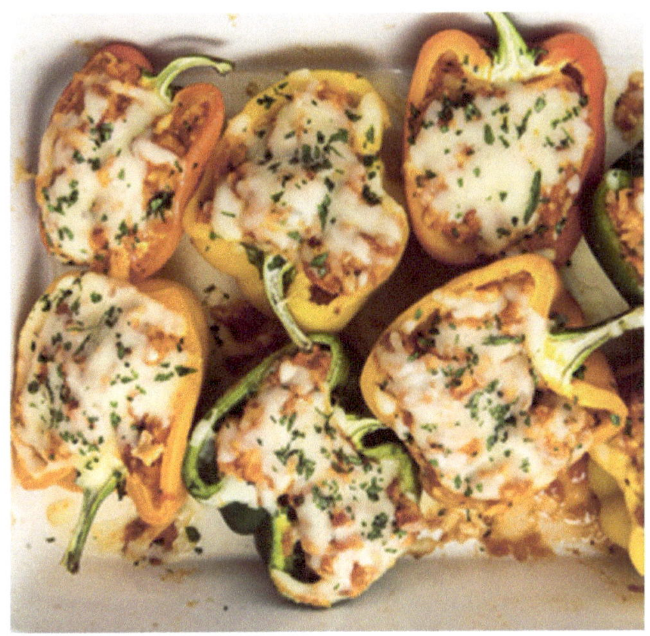

Serves 4

Ingredients

12 ounces frozen or fresh breaded chicken, cooked and diced

4 halved bell peppers with seeds removed

3 minced cloves of garlic

3 cups shredded and divided mozzarella

1 tablespoon freshly chopped parsley (plus more for garnishing)

1½ cups marinara

½ cup freshly grated Parmesan (plus more for serving)

½ cup chicken broth

Freshly ground black pepper

Kosher salt

Pinch of crushed red pepper flakes

Directions

1. Preheat your oven to 400°F.

2. In a large bowl, add red pepper flakes, parsley, marinara, garlic, parmesan and 2 cups of mozzarella. Season them with salt and pepper and stir well then gently fold in the chicken.

3. Spoon the mixture into the halved bell peppers and sprinkle with the remaining cup of mozzarella.

4. Add chicken broth into a baking dish and cover with foil to help the peppers to steam.

5. Put in the oven and bake for about 55 minutes or an hour until the peppers become tender.

6. Remove from oven and uncover thefoil then broil for 2 minutes

7. Garnish with parmesan and parsley then serve.

Baked Halibut

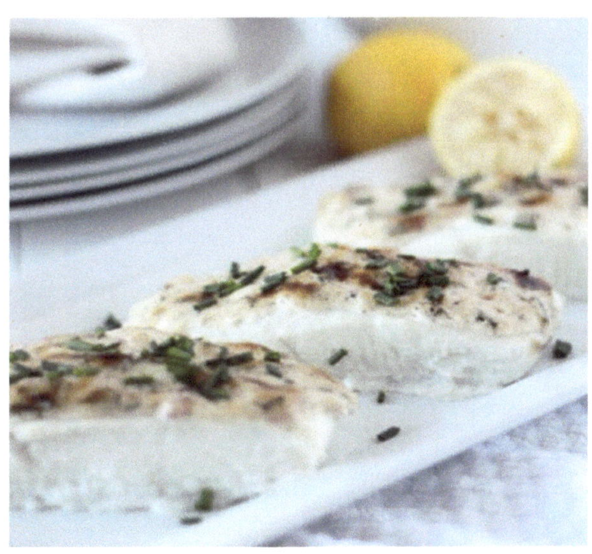

Serves 4

Ingredients

4 halibut fillets

2 tablespoons finely chopped chives

2 finely diced shallots

1 juiced lemon

1 tablespoon finely chopped parsley

1 teaspoon Dijon mustard

1/3 cup mayonnaise

¼ teaspoon pepper

Directions

1. Preheat your oven to 400°F.

2. In a small bowl, add half of the chives (the other half is for garnishing), mustard, mayonnaise, pepper and lemon juice and stir.

3. Coat the inside of a baking dish lightly with butter or oil to prevent the halibut form sticking. Place the fillets in the dish.

4. Spoon the mayonnaise mixture evenly onto the top of the halibut fillets and bake for 15 to 20 minutes. Be careful to avoid overcooking.

5. Just before the fish is done, turn on the top broiler of the oven for 1 or 2 minutes. You will know the fish is done when it becomes opaque.

6. Remove it from the oven and sprinkle the rest of the chives on top then serve while hot with some rice and green vegetables.

Honey Garlic Glazed Salmon

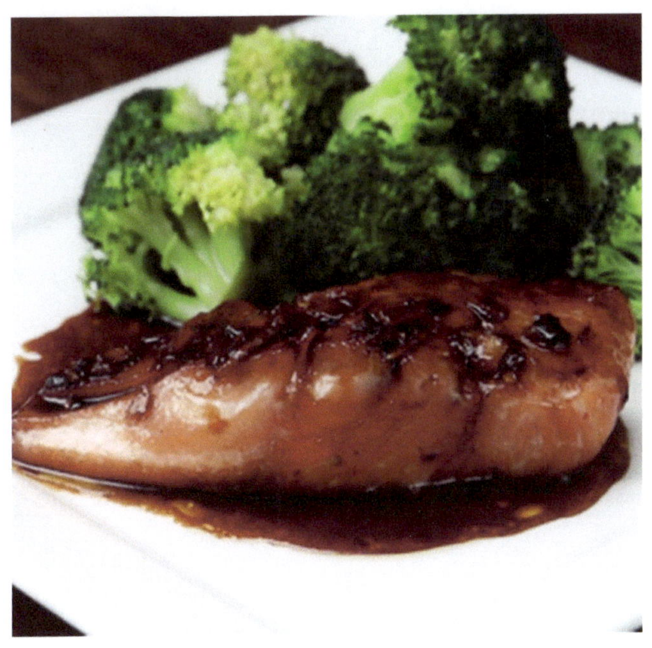

Serves 4

Ingredients

4 salmon fillets (patted dry with paper towels)

3 minced cloves of garlic

3 tablespoons extra virgin oil

2 tablespoons lemon juice

Freshly chopped parsley

Freshly ground black pepper

Kosher salt

1 round-sliced lemon pieces

1 teaspoon red pepper flakes

¼ cup of soy sauce

1/3 cup of honey

Directions

1. Whisk together lemon juice, soy sauce, honey and red pepper flakes in a medium bowl

2. In a skillet over medium-high heat, heat 2 tablespoons of oil.

3. Add the salmon fillet with the skin side up and season with salt and pepper.

4. Cook for about 6 minutes until it turns deep golden then flip over and add a tablespoon of oil.

5. Add garlic and cook for a minute until fragrant. Throw in the sliced lemons and honey mixture and cook until the sauce reduces by about a third. Baste the salmon with the sauce.

6. Garnish with parsley and sliced lemon then serve with some broccoli.

Osso Bucco with Soft Polenta

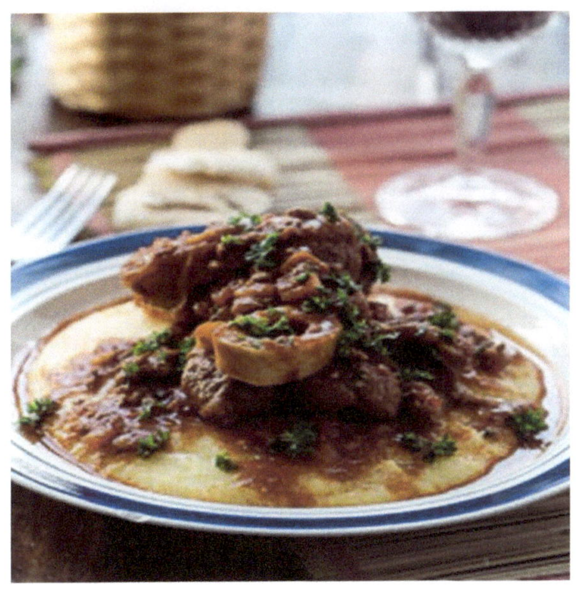

Serves 4

Ingredients

4 Osso Bucco beef steaks

2 minced or crushed cloves of garlic

2 diced carrots

1 tablespoon vegetable stock powder

1 can of condensed either crushed tomatoes, tomato soup or pasta sauce

1 tablespoon tomato paste

1 finely chopped onion

1 tablespoon garlic olive oil

¼ cup dry red wine

¼ cup of water

Polenta, prepared depending on package instructions

Parsley

Salt to taste

Directions

1. Heat oil in a large frying pan and add the onions, garlic and carrots. Cook until onion turns transparent.

2. Add the Osso Bucco steaks and brown both sides.

3. Add soup or paste sauce, wine, tomato paste, water and stock powder.

4. Reduce heat, cover and let it simmer for 1 to 1½ hours until beef is tender.

5. Season with some salt and serve this over prepared polenta and garnish with some parsley.

Avocado Chickpea Tuna Salad

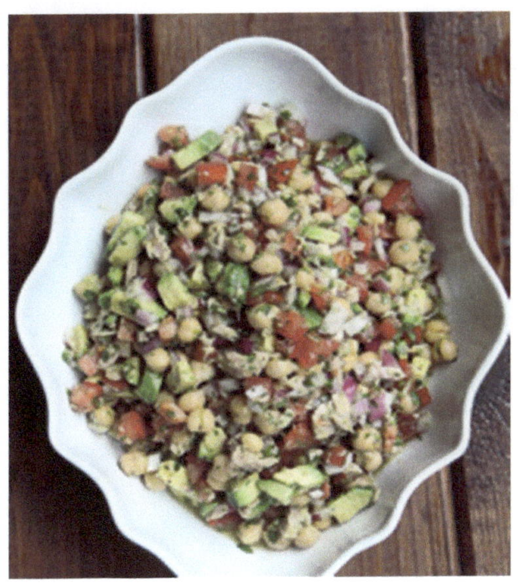

Serves 4

Ingredients for the dressing

2 tablespoons freshly squeezed lemon juice

1 teaspoon minced garlic

1 tablespoon freshly chopped parsley (plus extra for serving)

¼ teaspoon salt

¼ cup olive oil

Ingredients for the salad

15 ounces canned tuna (canned in olive oil or brine)

14 ounces can of chickpeas, drained

2 large wedge-cut tomatoes

2 large peeled and pitted avocadoes

1 large cucumber, halved lengthwise and sliced

½ thinly sliced red onion

Directions

1. Put all the dressing ingredients in a jar or jug and whisk them together.

2. Mix the salad ingredients together in a large bowl. Toss the dressing on top.

3. Season with pepper and salt.

Beef Salad

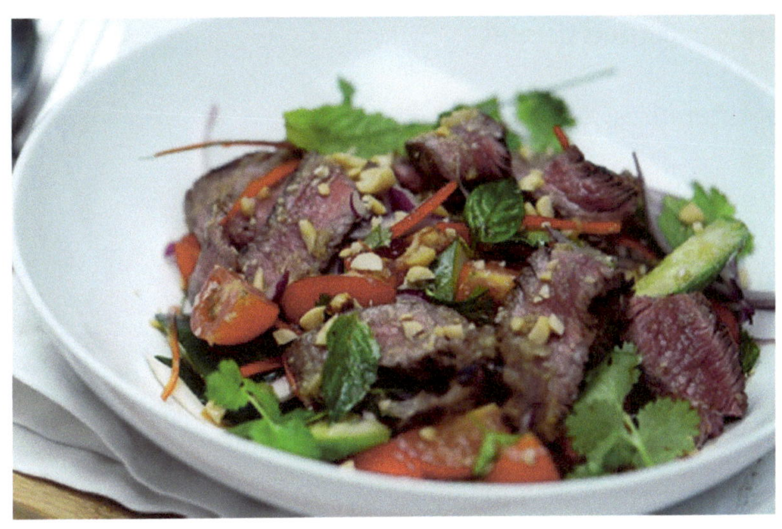

Serves 1

Ingredients

½ tablespoon tamari soybean sauce

½ garlic clove

¼ teaspoon sesame oil

¼ tablespoon sodium and sugar free rice vinegar

1/8 teaspoon curry powder

1/8 teaspoon sucralose based sweetener

1/16 teaspoon ginger

¾ cup spring mix salad

4 ¼ oz. beef top sirloin

¼ large sweet red pepper

2 oz. water chestnuts

1 large scallion/ spring onion

½ tablespoon canola vegetable oil

Directions

1. In a small bowl, mix green onions, soy sauce, sesame oil, rice wine vinegar, and sugar substitute.

2. Pour the mixture into a re-sealable plastic bag.

3. Add steak into the bag and marinate in the fridge overnight.

4. Add ginger and curry powder to the remaining soy mixture.

5. In a large skillet, heat canola oil over high heat until very hot.

6. Drain the marinated beef and discard the marinade. Stir-fry the beef for approximately 2-3 minutes in the hot oil, and then transfer to a large mixing bowl.

7. Add bell pepper, salad greens, reserved soy dressing and water chestnuts into the bowl and toss to coat.

Frequently Asked Questions (FAQS) About Intermittent Fasting

This chapter will answer some questions you may have about intermittent fasting

1. Is it not unhealthy to skip breakfast?

Contrary to popular belief, breakfast is not the most important meal. Skipping it when fasting actually can present you with many health benefits such as burning more fat to produce energy as well as improving insulin sensitivity.

2. Is it true that fasting slows down metabolism?

Not really. Recent <u>studies</u> suggest that fasting in the long term in reality boosts your metabolism. However it is not such a good idea to extend the fasting period for too long.

3. Is it true that fasting can catabolize muscles?

Not at all. You may even fast for as long as 40 hours without stimulating the catabolic processes that leads to skeletal muscle atrophy. In fact, if you consume any meal containing proteins within 1 or 2 days of a resistance training session, your muscles will grow bigger.

4. Why is it advisable to drink coffee during a fast?

Coffee actually plays a part in fat burning. This study found that epinephrine (a hormone whose production is stimulated by coffee) augments thermogenic and lipolytic effects. In simple terms this means that fat breakdown and metabolism all increase considerably after epinephrine is produced. Epinephrine also lowers appetite so you won't have to worry about going for a long fasting period.

5. Are children allowed to fast?

Absolutely not!! Children should not be put under a fasting regimen until they become adults

6. Out of all those fasting protocols, which one is the best?

All are equal. There isn't the best or the worst protocol but the more intense protocols tend to give you quick results. Some people would prefer to take it slow while others need fast results.

Conclusion

We have come to the end of the book. Thank you for reading and congratulations for reading until the end.

While research on intermittent fasting may still be in its formative years, you cannot overlook the effectiveness of intermittent fasting. Furthermore, you can improve the effectiveness of intermittent fasting by exercising while in a fasted state and drinking plenty of water and coffee and tea without milk or sugar. When it is time to eat, focus on healthy foods rather than binging on junk food, and you will be amazed at how much weight you can lose.

If you found the book valuable, can you recommend it to others? One way to do that is to post a review on Amazon.

Click here to leave a review for this book on Amazon!

Thank you and good luck!